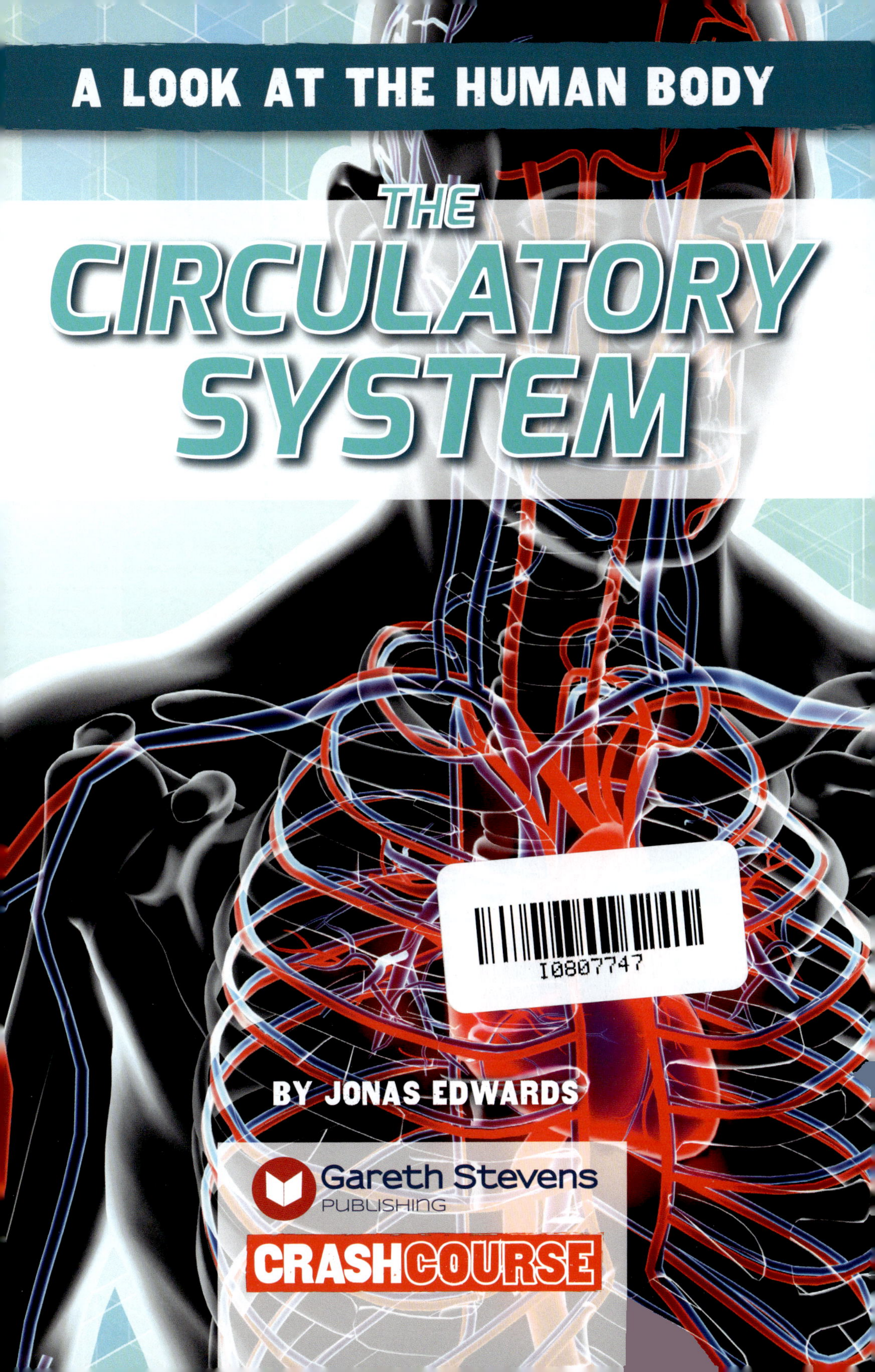

A LOOK AT THE HUMAN BODY

THE CIRCULATORY SYSTEM

BY JONAS EDWARDS

Gareth Stevens PUBLISHING

CRASHCOURSE

Please visit our website, www.garethstevens.com. For a free color catalog of all our high-quality books, call toll free 1-800-542-2595 or fax 1-877-542-2596.

Library of Congress Cataloging-in-Publication Data

Names: Edwards, Jonas, author.
Title: The circulatory system / Jonas Edwards.
Description: New York : Gareth Stevens Publishing, [2022] | Series: A look at the human body | Includes index.
Identifiers: LCCN 2020013443 | ISBN 9781538266076 (library binding) | ISBN 9781538266052 (paperback) | ISBN 9781538266069 (6 pack) | ISBN 9781538266083 (ebook)
Subjects: LCSH: Cardiovascular system—Juvenile literature.
Classification: LCC QM178 .E39 2022 | DDC 612.1—dc23
LC record available at https://lccn.loc.gov/2020013443

First Edition

Published in 2022 by
Gareth Stevens Publishing
29 E. 21st Street
New York, NY 10010

Editor: Kate Mikoley
Designer: Andrea Davison-Bartolotta

Photo credits: Cover MDGRPHCS/Shutterstock.com; background texture Yuliia Petrenko/Shutterstock.com; p. 5 (top) Catherine Delahaye/Stone/Getty Images; p. 5 (bottom) Westend61/Getty Images; pp. 7 (top), 21 Science Photo Library – Pixologic Studio/Brand X Pictures/Getty Images; p. 7 (bottom) Jonathan Kitchen/The Image Bank/Getty Images; p. 9 (top) posteriori/E+/Getty Images; p. 9 (bottom) SCIEPRO/Science Photo Library/Getty Images; p. 11 (top) FatCamera/E+/Getty Images; p. 11 (bottom) adventtr/E+/Getty Images; p. 13 (main) colematt/iStock/Getty Images Plus/Getty Images; pp. 13 (background), 15 (background), 19 (background) Olga OleNN/Shutterstock.com; p. 15 (main) Marochkina Anastasiia/Shutterstock.com; p. 17 kali9/iStock/Getty Images Plus/Getty Images; p. 19 (heart) Designua/Shutterstock.com; p. 19 (door) Scott Van Dyke/Corbis Documentary/Getty Images; p. 23 mustafagull/E+/Getty Images; p. 25 (top) Marie Schmitt/Corbis Documentary/Getty Images Plus/Getty Images; p. 25 (bottom) Inok/iStock/Getty Images Plus/Getty Images; p. 27 Sebastian Kaulitzki/Science Photo Library/Getty Images; p. 29 (top) Jose Luis Pelaez Inc./DigitalVision/Getty Images; p. 29 (bottom) Rolf Bruderer/Getty Images; p. 30 (heart) Rendix Alextian/Shutterstock.com.

Printed in the United States of America

Some of the images in this book illustrate individuals who are models. The depictions do not imply actual situations or events.

CPSIA compliance information: Batch #CSGS22: For further information contact Gareth Stevens, New York, New York at 1-800-542-2595.

CONTENTS

Words in the glossary appear in **bold** type the first time they are used in the text.

STAYING ALIVE

You likely know that you need **oxygen** and nutrients to live. But how do these things get around your body? They travel in your blood as part of your circulatory system! Read on to learn how this bodily system works.

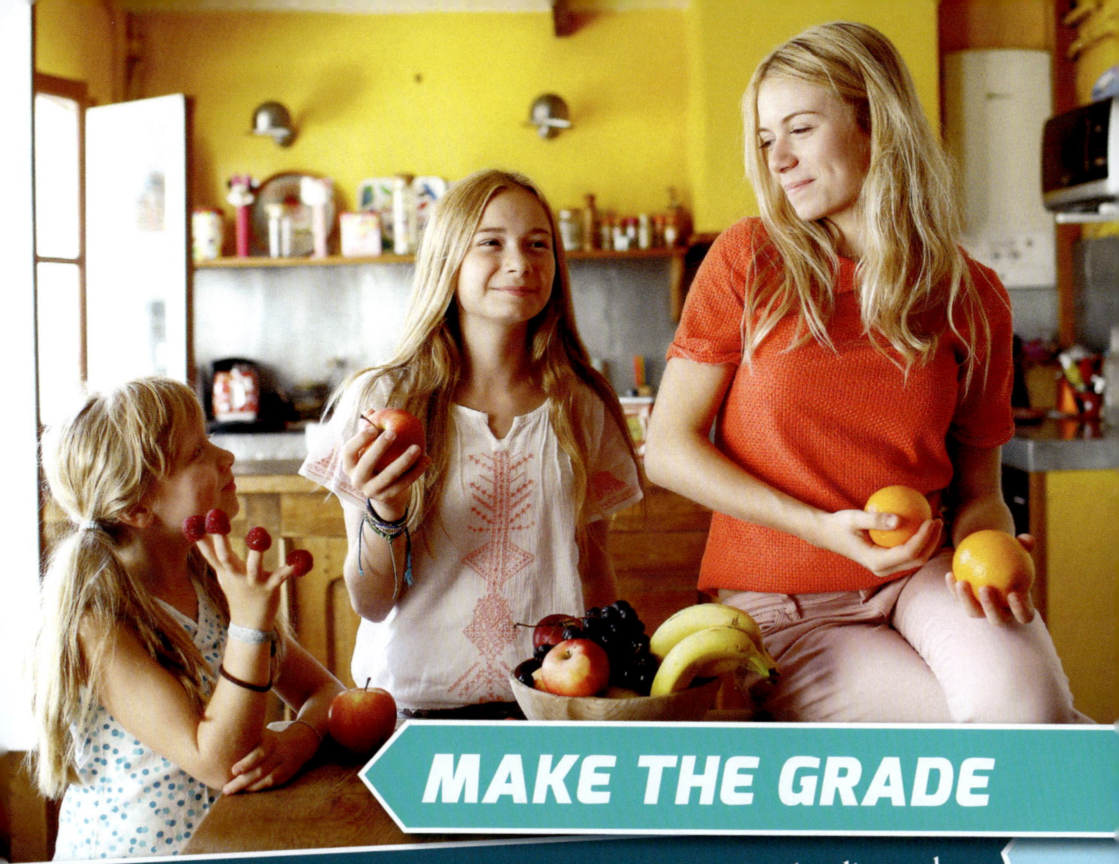

MAKE THE GRADE

Nutrients are things that living things—like you!—need to live and grow. Nutrients can come into your body through the foods you eat.

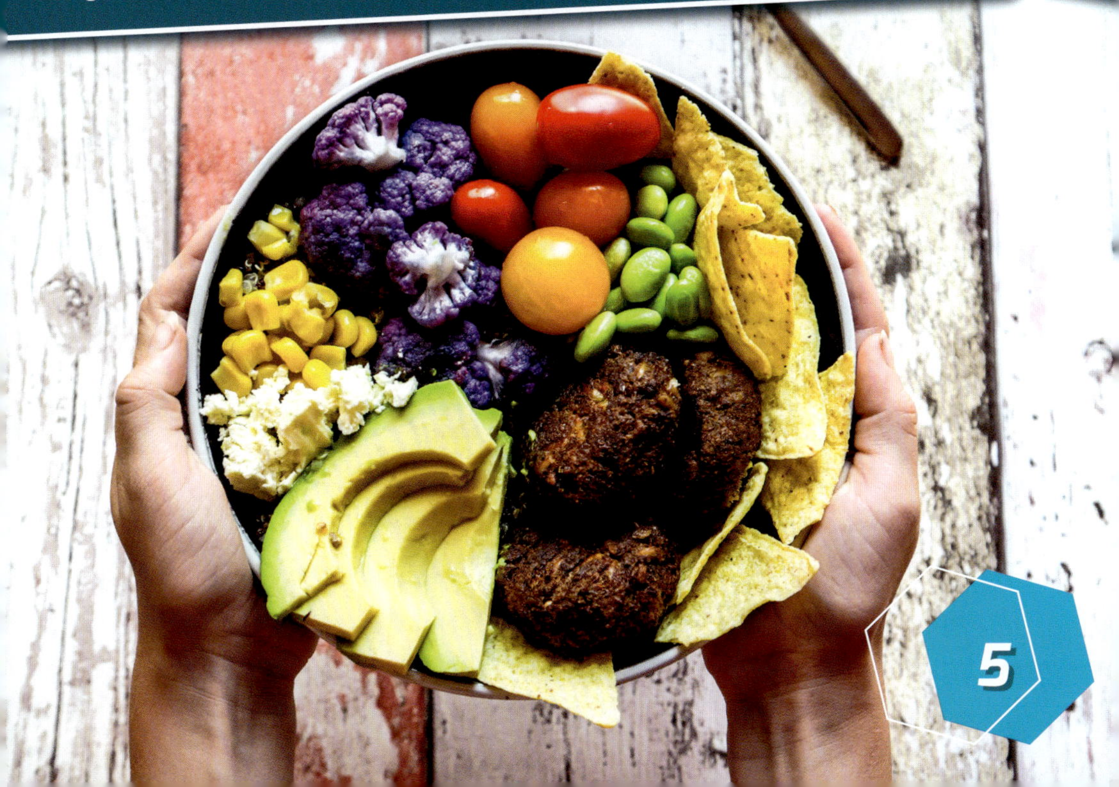

BLOOD FLOWS!

The human circulatory system is made up of the heart, blood, and blood vessels. Every time your heart beats, it sends blood through your body. Blood vessels are small **tubes** that carry this blood away from and back toward the heart.

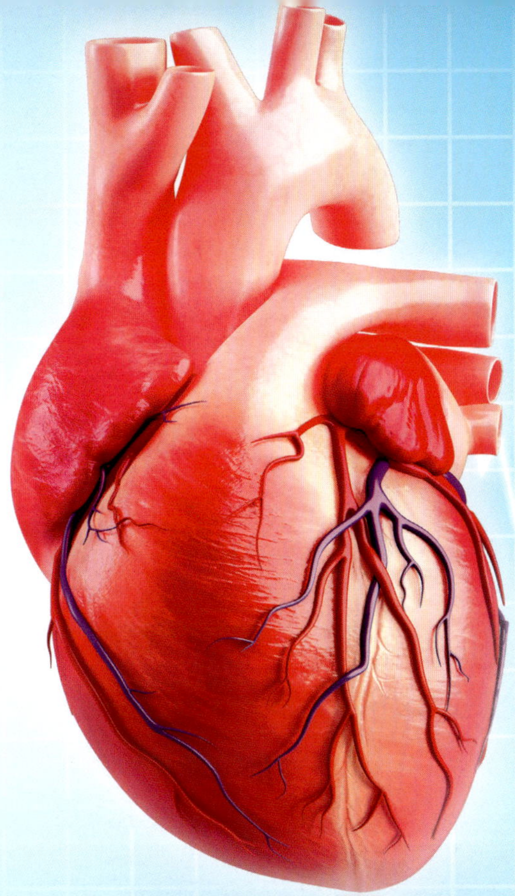

MAKE THE GRADE

When blood moves through the heart and around the body, it's called circulation. This is where the name "circulatory system" comes from.

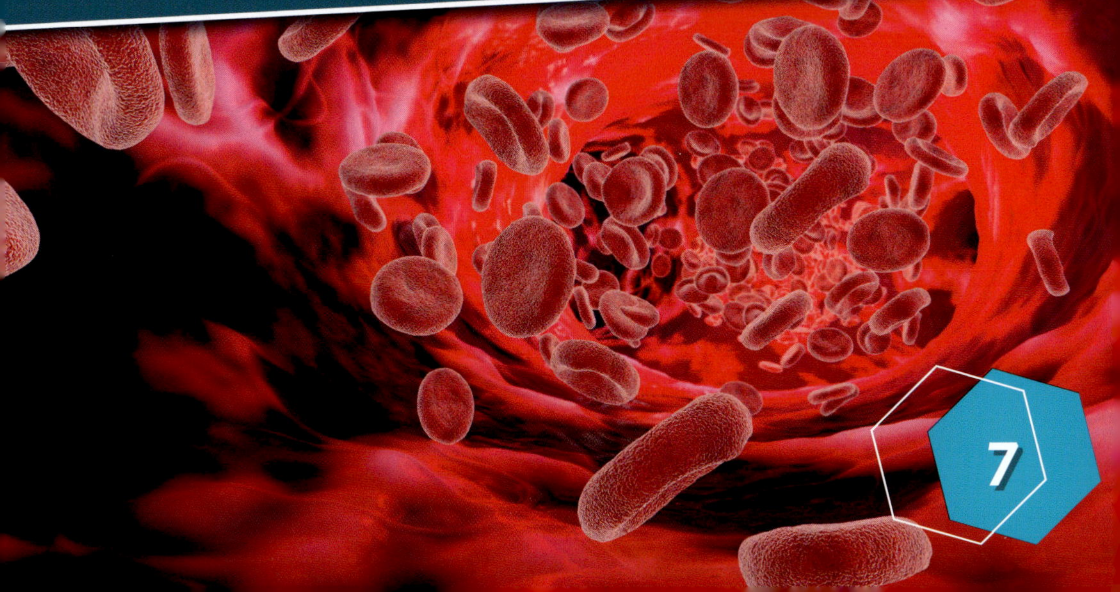

Arteries are the blood vessels that carry blood away from the heart. The blood vessels that carry blood from other parts of the body back to the heart are called veins. The smallest blood vessels are called capillaries.

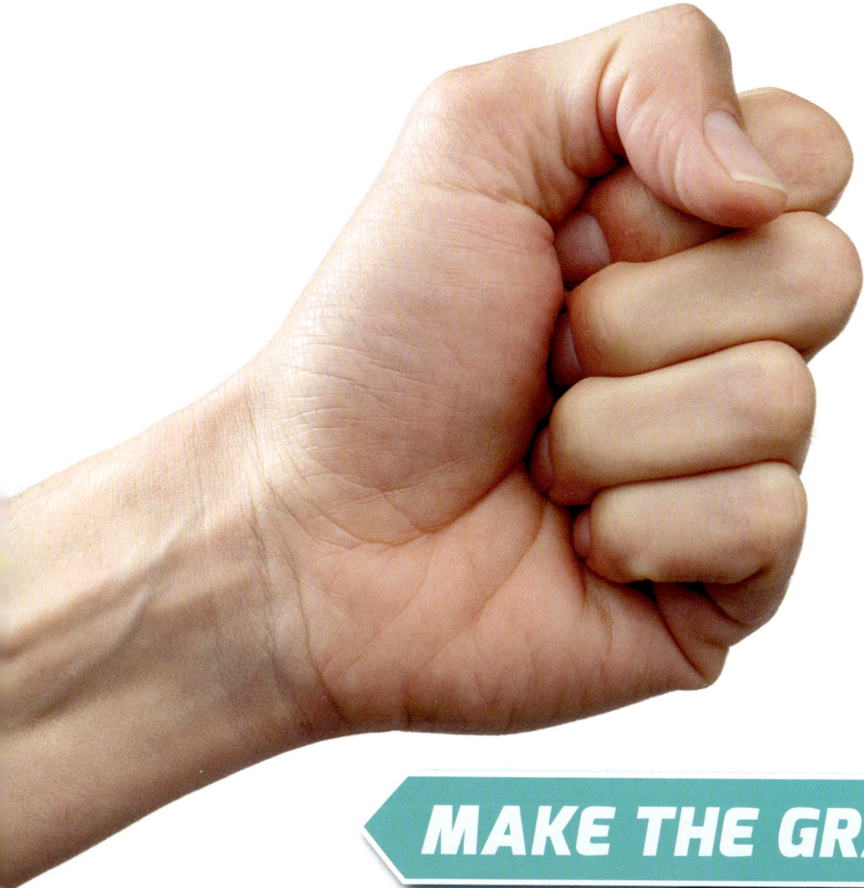

MAKE THE GRADE

Your heart is a **muscle**! It's about the same size as a closed fist.

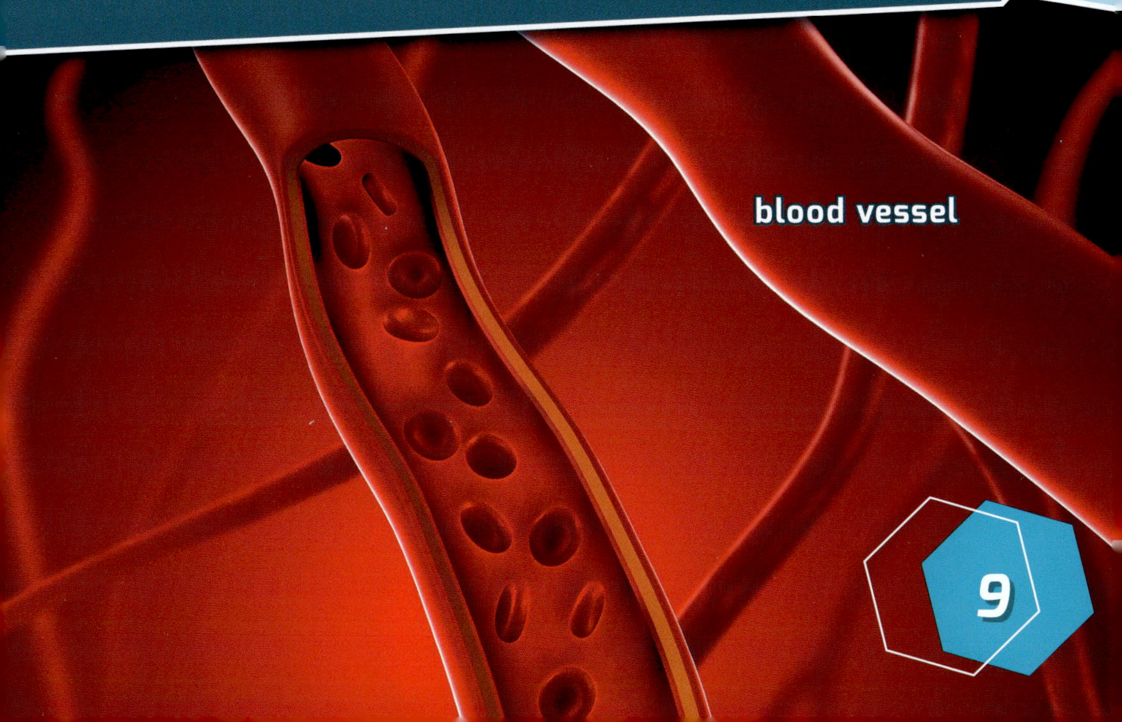

TAKING SIDES

Each side of the heart has a different job. The right side takes in blood from the body and sends it out to the **lungs**. The left side takes in blood from the lungs and sends it out to the rest of the body.

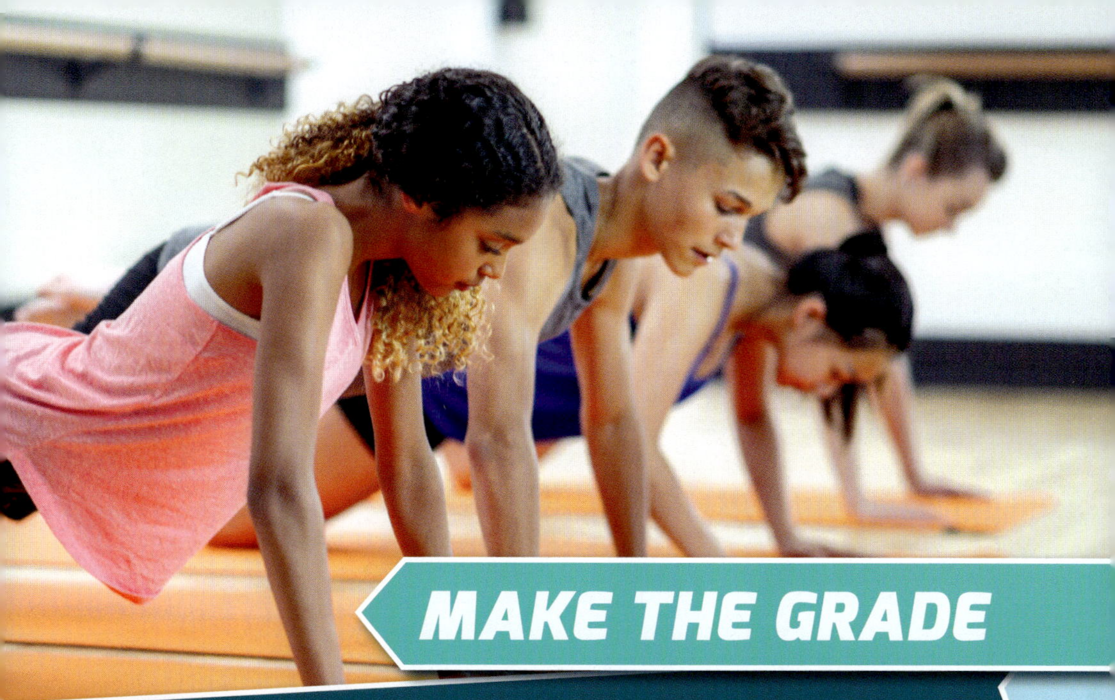

MAKE THE GRADE

It takes less than a minute for your circulatory system to send blood to every cell in your body!

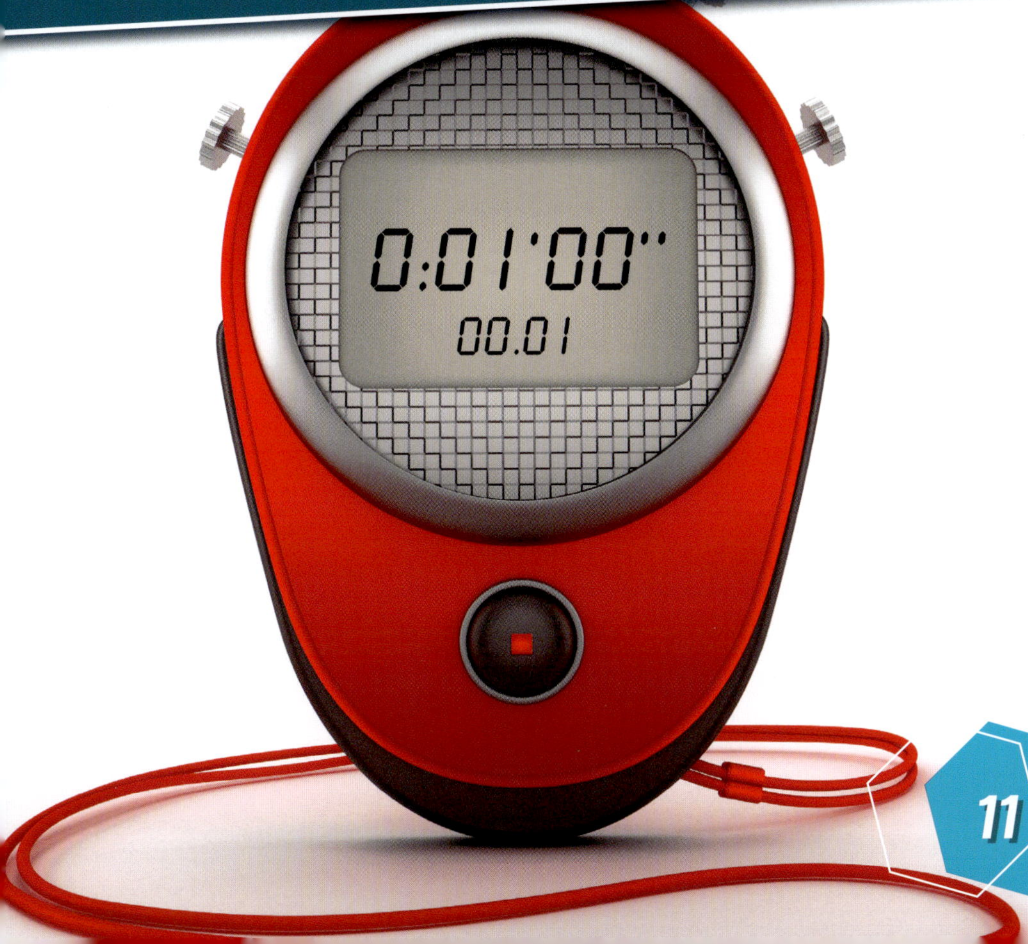

CHAMBERS OF THE HEART

The heart has four main parts, or chambers. The top two chambers are called the atria. When you're talking about only one of these two chambers, it's called an atrium. Each atrium takes in blood coming back to the heart.

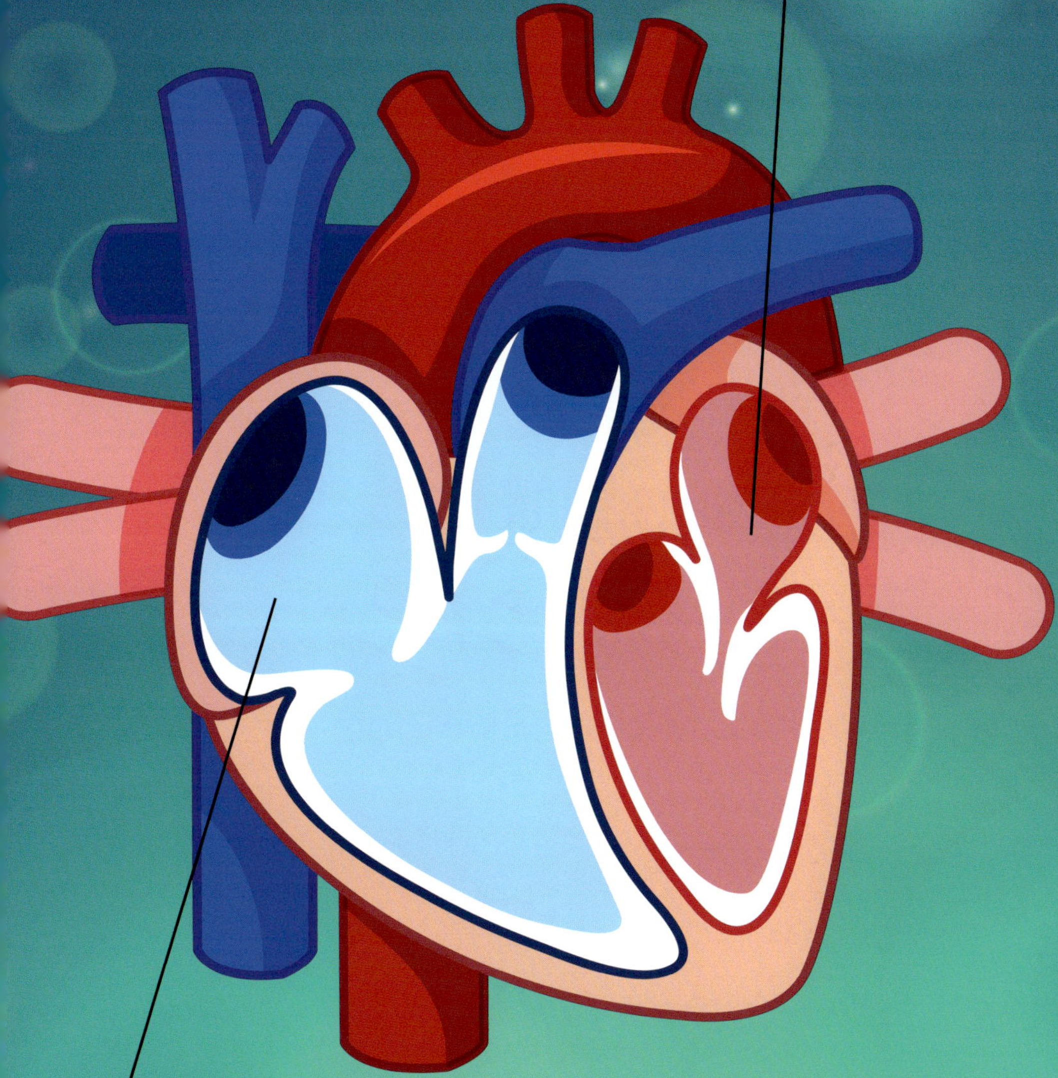

MAKE THE GRADE

The right atrium takes in blood returning from the body. The left atrium takes in blood returning from the lungs.

The heart's bottom two chambers are the ventricles. These chambers send the blood out. The right ventricle sends blood out to the lungs, while the left ventricle sends it out to the rest of the body.

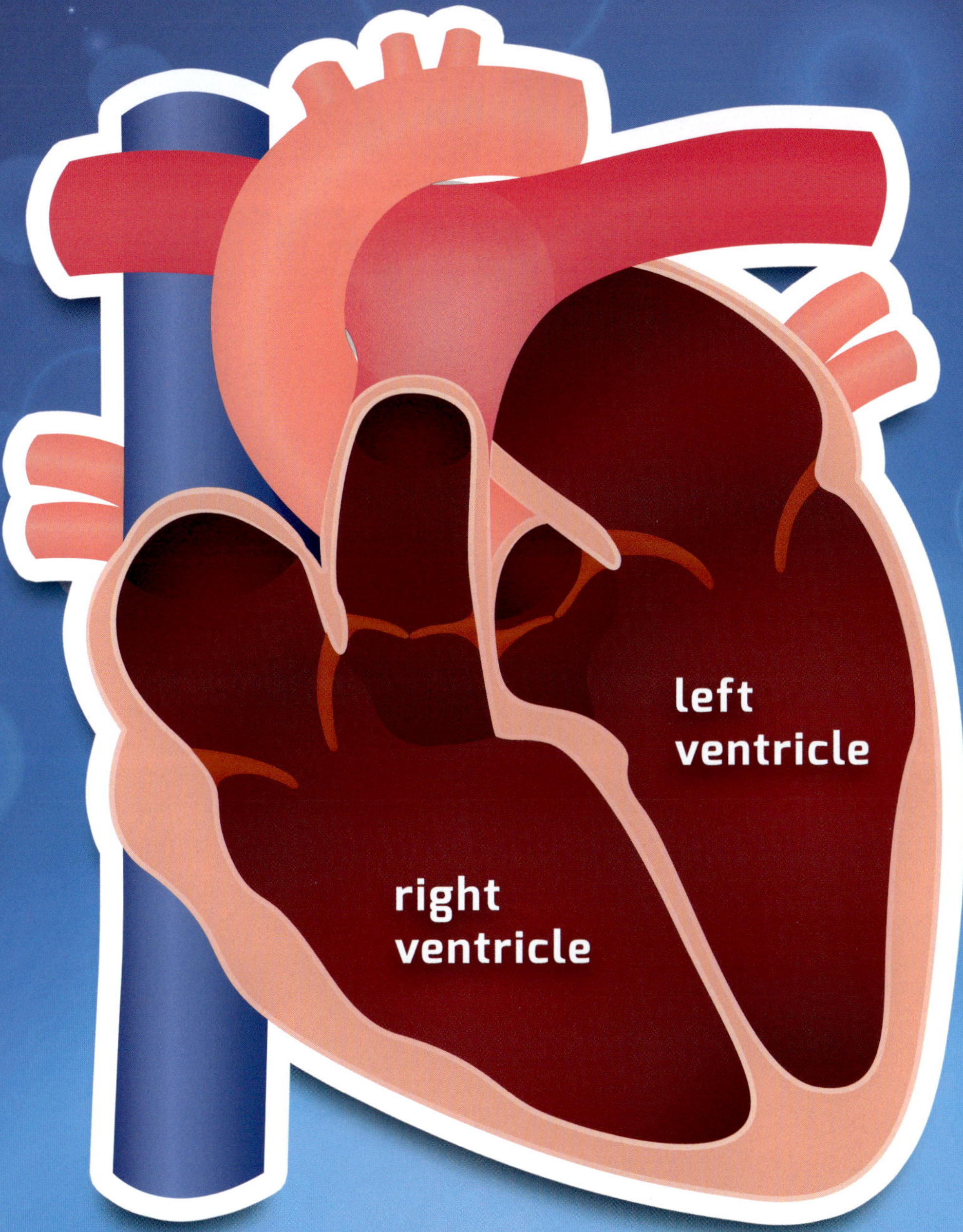

MAKE THE GRADE

Most of the force for **pumping** blood comes from the ventricles. As a result, the walls of the ventricles have more muscle than the walls of the atria.

A TEAM EFFORT

The atria and ventricles have to work together. As the ventricles **contract** and send the blood out of the heart, the atria fill with more blood. Then, they pass this blood along to the ventricles so the **cycle** can continue.

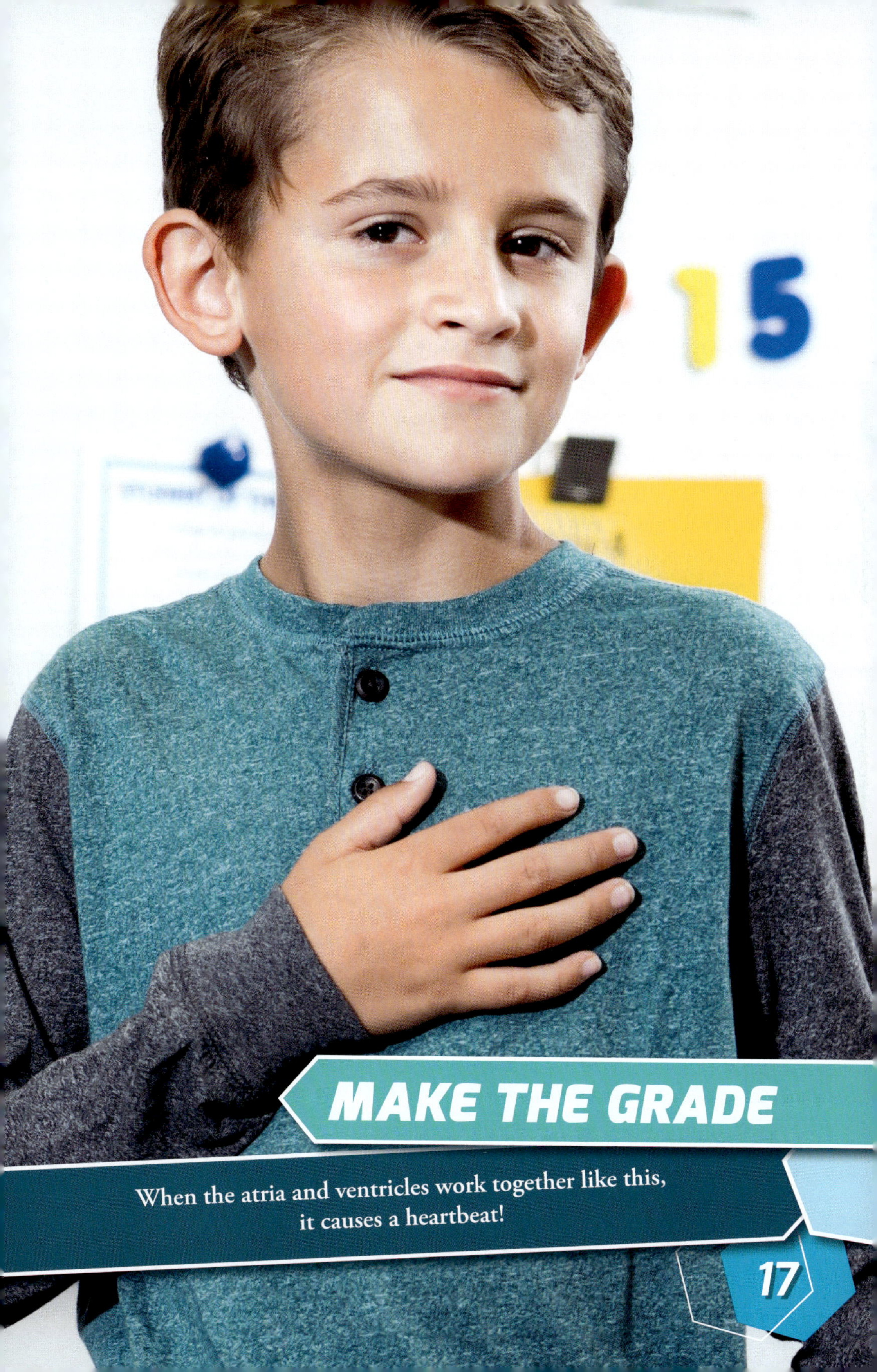

MAKE THE GRADE

When the atria and ventricles work together like this, it causes a heartbeat!

MOVING ALONG

The chambers of the heart are separated by **valves.** Valves make sure that the blood flows only in the proper direction. The two valves that allow blood to move from the atria to the ventricles are called the mitral and tricuspid valves.

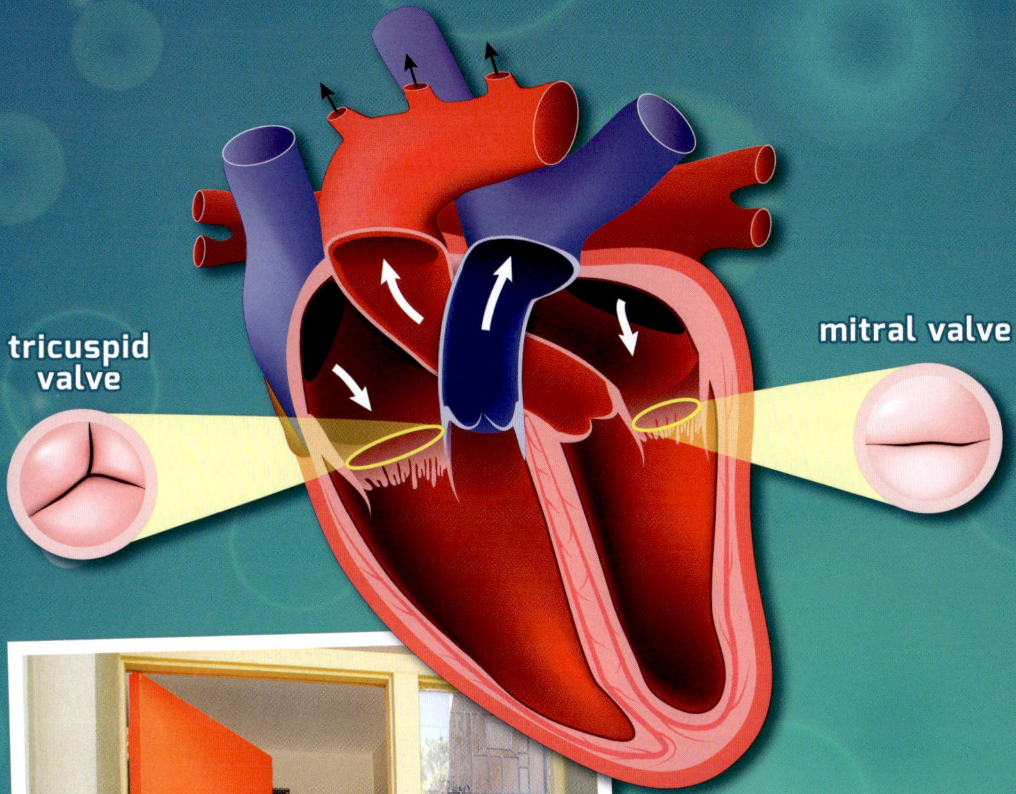

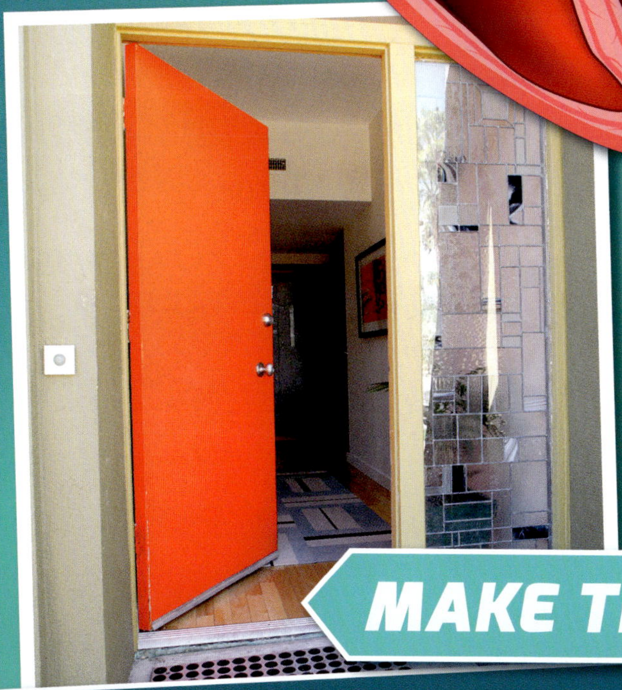

MAKE THE GRADE

Valves can open and close like a door. The mitral valve goes between the left atrium and the left ventricle. The tricuspid valve goes between the right atrium and the right ventricle.

The aorta is the blood vessel that carries blood from the heart to the rest of the body. The aortic valve is between the left ventricle and aorta. The pulmonary valve is between the right ventricle and the pulmonary artery, which brings blood to the lungs.

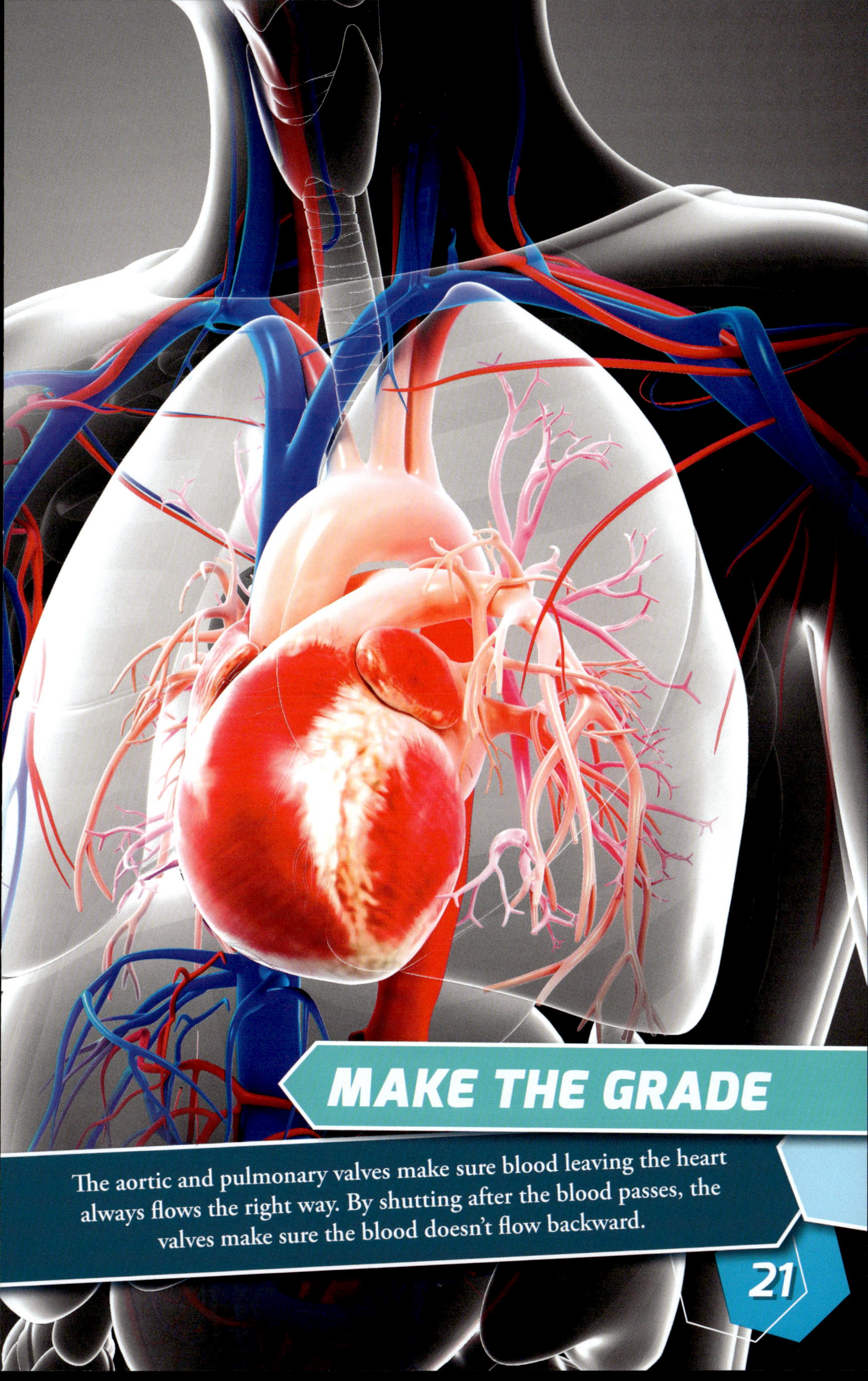

MAKE THE GRADE

The aortic and pulmonary valves make sure blood leaving the heart always flows the right way. By shutting after the blood passes, the valves make sure the blood doesn't flow backward.

PULMONARY CIRCULATION

Blood takes two different paths during circulation. Pulmonary circulation is when blood makes its way from the heart to the lungs, through the pulmonary valve and artery. It returns back to the heart through the pulmonary veins.

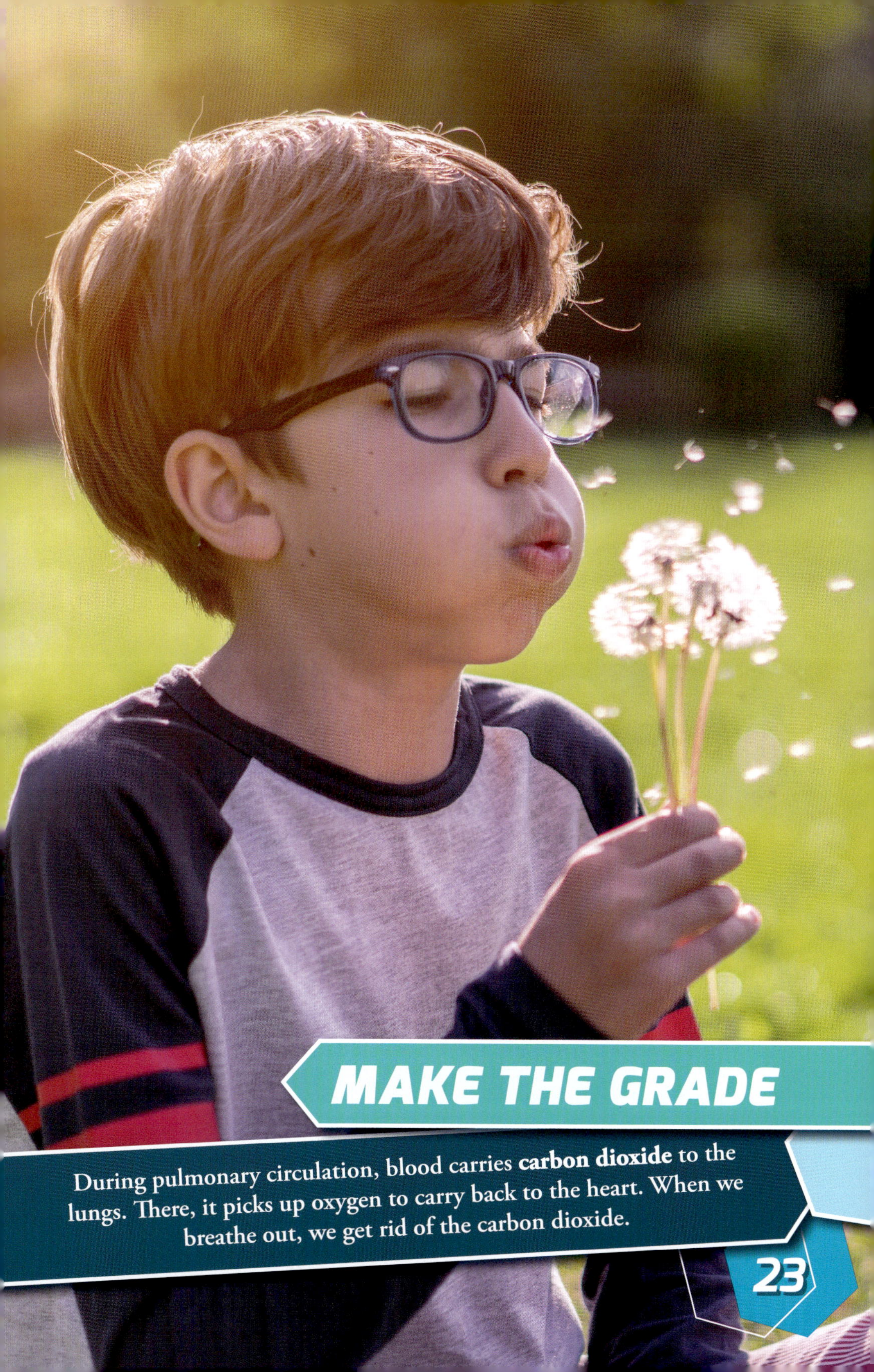

MAKE THE GRADE

During pulmonary circulation, blood carries **carbon dioxide** to the lungs. There, it picks up oxygen to carry back to the heart. When we breathe out, we get rid of the carbon dioxide.

SYSTEMIC CIRCULATION

After pulmonary circulation, systemic circulation takes over. The blood, now full of oxygen breathed in and picked up from the lungs, is sent to the rest of the body through the aorta. Small branches stem from the aorta, taking blood to other body parts.

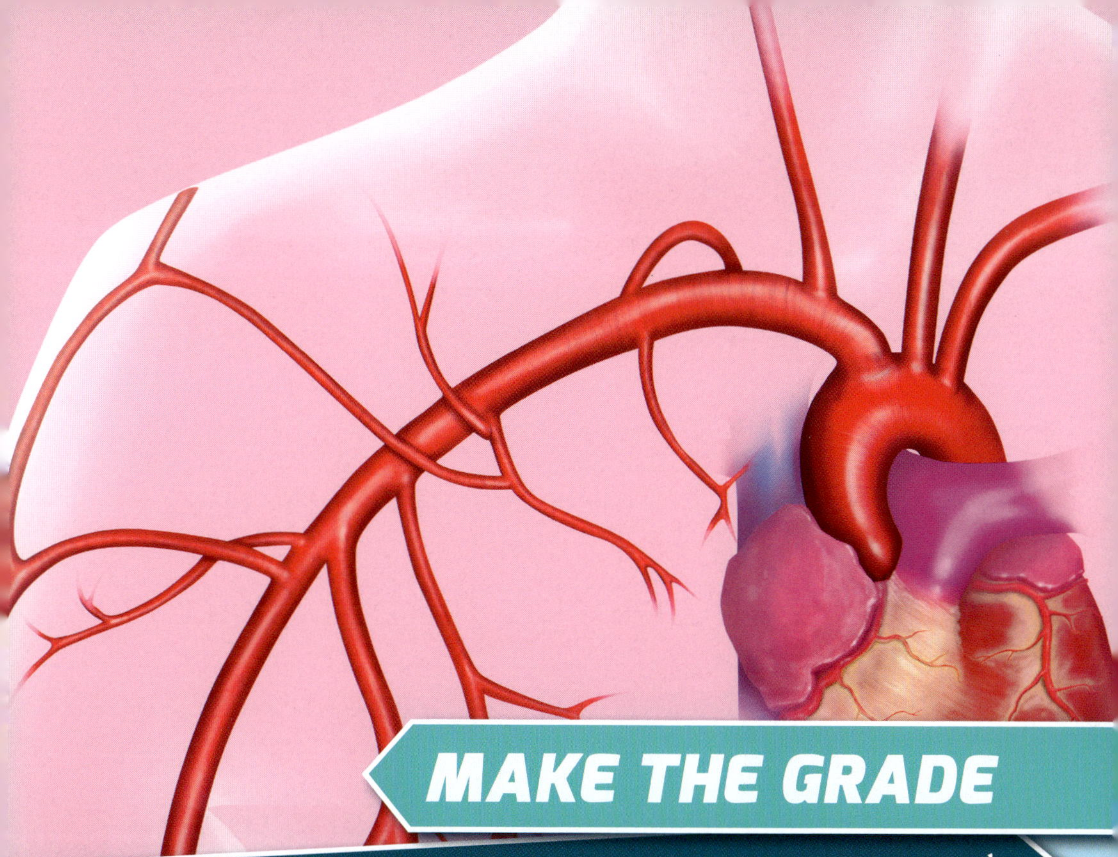

MAKE THE GRADE

Artery branches are connected to small veins by capillaries. Nutrients and oxygen pass through the capillaries' thin walls and are delivered to the cells.

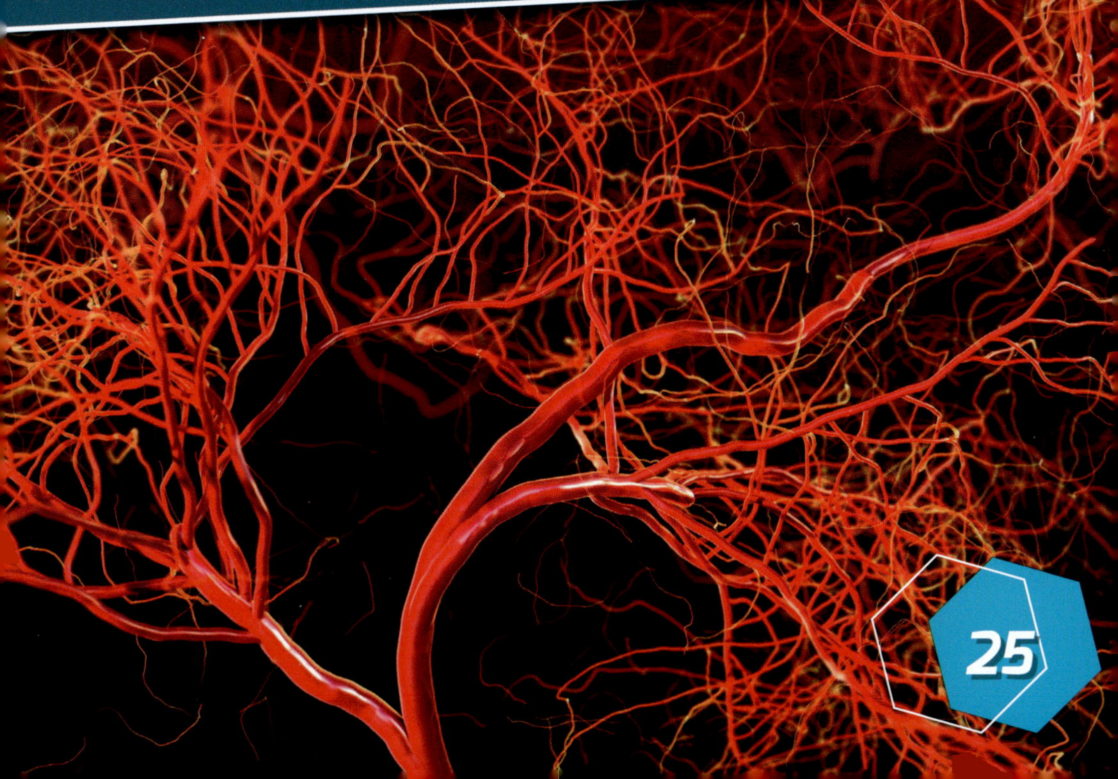

In the veins, valves keep the blood moving in the correct direction. The closer the blood gets to the heart, the larger the veins are. Once the blood returns to the heart, it's time to start pulmonary circulation again.

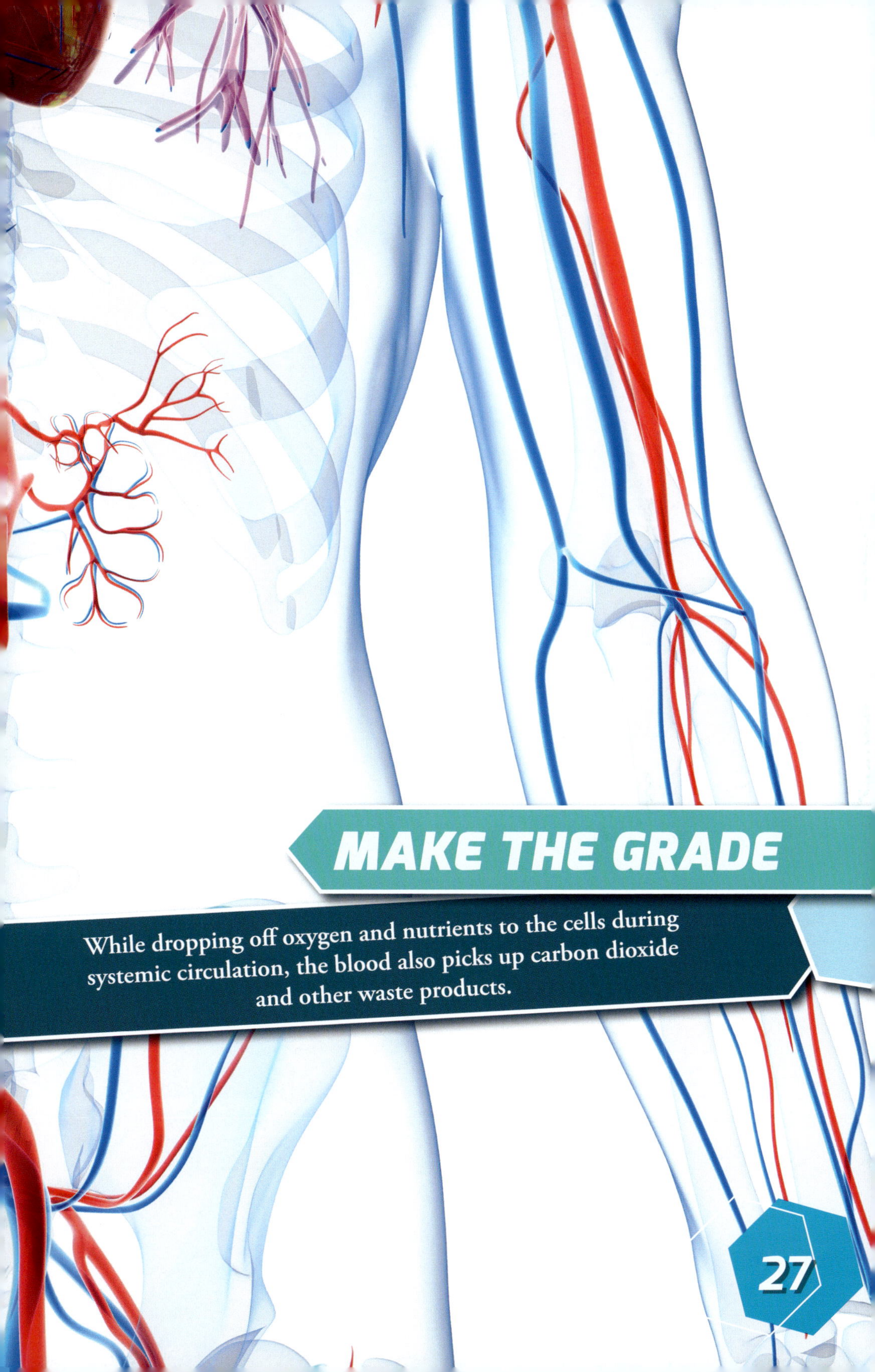

MAKE THE GRADE

While dropping off oxygen and nutrients to the cells during systemic circulation, the blood also picks up carbon dioxide and other waste products.

CIRCULATION SOUNDS

Doctors use a tool called a stethoscope to listen to your heart. It sounds like "lub-dub." The closing of the mitral and tricuspid valves makes the "lub" sound. The "dub" sound happens as the aortic and pulmonary valves close.

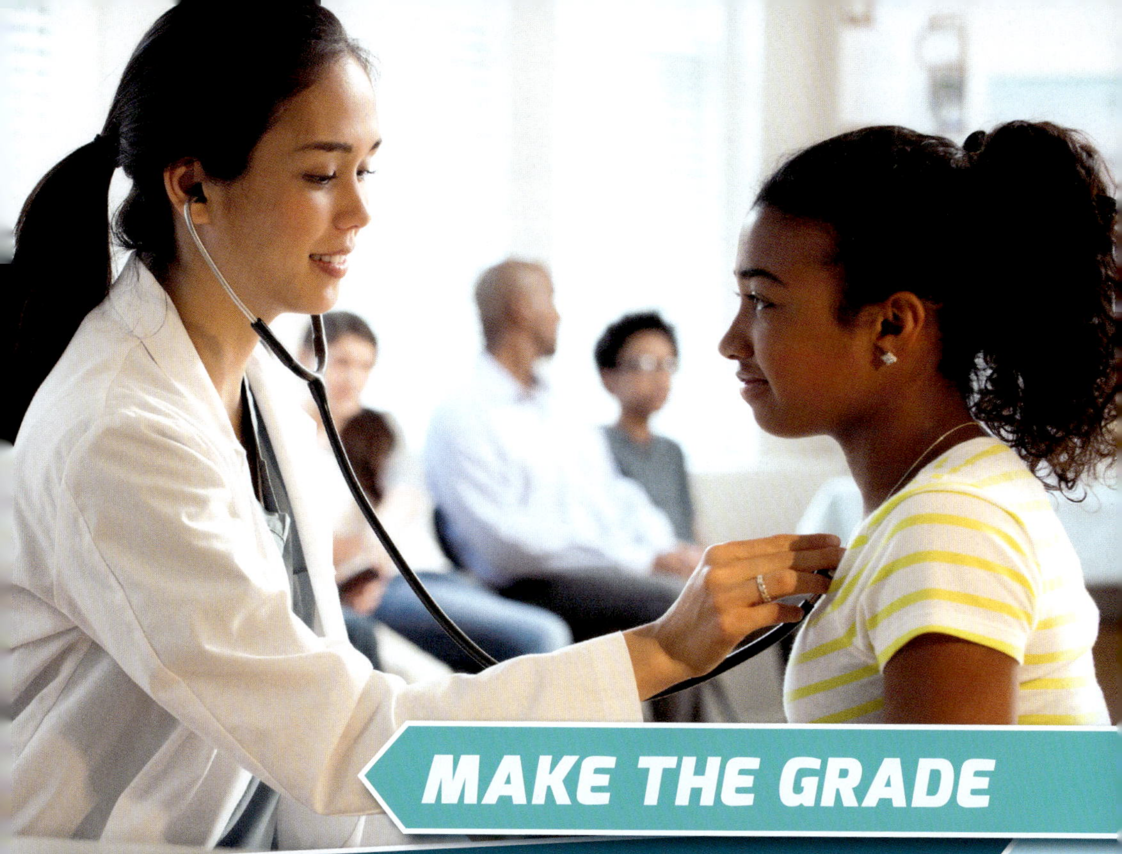

MAKE THE GRADE

Keep your circulatory system in great shape by keeping your heart healthy. One way to do this is to move in ways that get you breathing heavy, like dancing or jumping rope.

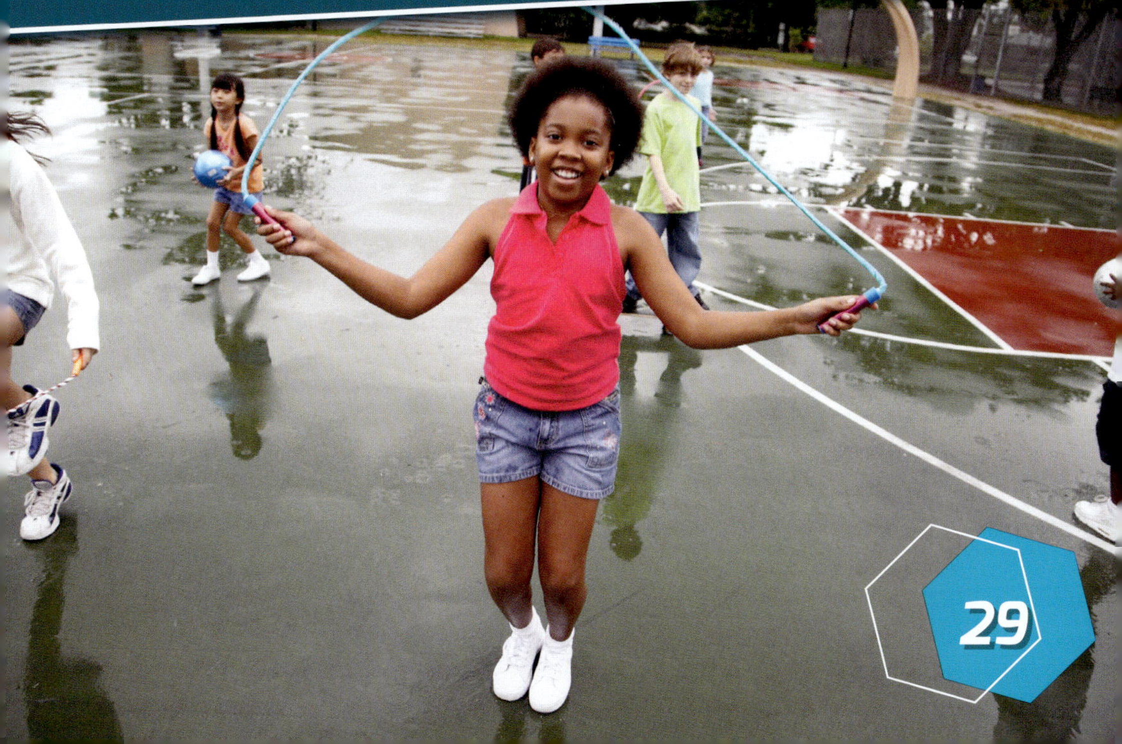

PARTS OF THE HEART

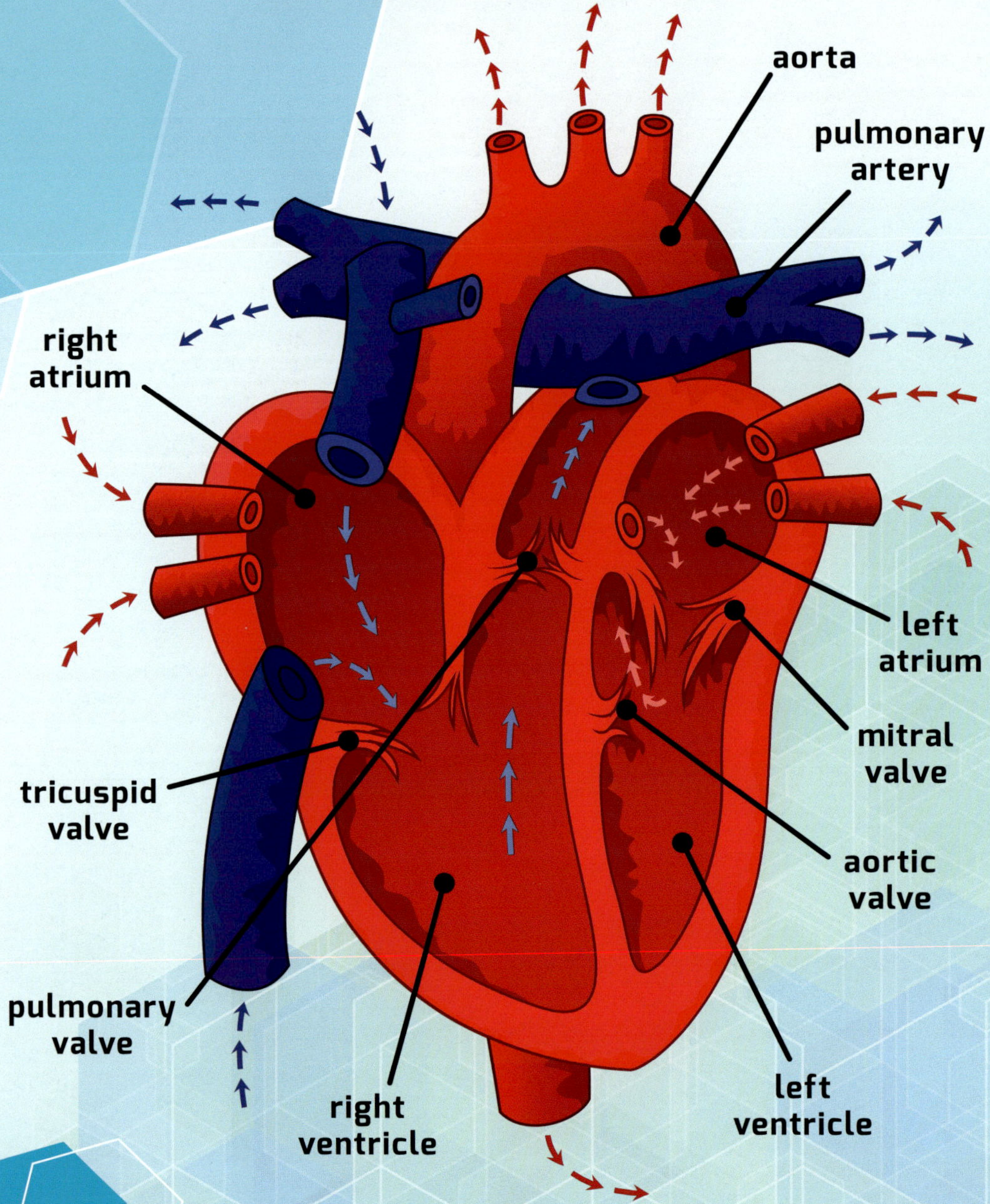

GLOSSARY

carbon dioxide: a gas breathed out by animals

contract: to get smaller and tighter

cycle: a sequence of events that repeats

lung: a part of an animal that takes in air when it breathes

muscle: one of the parts of the body that allow movement

oxygen: a colorless, odorless gas that many animals, including people, need to breathe

pump: to force a liquid, such as blood, to move through a tube or vessel

tube: a thin, long, hollow part of an animal that liquid, such as blood, or gas can flow through

valve: a part that opens and closes, allowing fluid to move in only one direction

FOR MORE INFORMATION

BOOKS

Farndon, John. *Stickmen's Guide to Your Beating Heart.* Minneapolis, MN: Hungry Tomato, 2018.

Rustad, Martha E. H. *My Circulatory System: A 4D Book.* North Mankato, MN: Pebble, 2019.

WEBSITES

Heart
www.dkfindout.com/us/human-body/heart-and-blood/heart/
Head to this website to learn more about this central part of the circulatory system.

Your Heart and Circulatory System
kidshealth.org/en/kids/heart.html
Find more fascinating facts about the circulatory system on this website.

Publisher's note to educators and parents: Our editors have carefully reviewed these websites to ensure that they are suitable for students. Many websites change frequently, however, and we cannot guarantee that a site's future contents will continue to meet our high standards of quality and educational value. Be advised that students should be closely supervised whenever they access the internet.

INDEX